Low Carb Diet For Beginners

A Complete Compilation Of All The Tips To Low Carb, High Fat Diet, The Winning Formula To Lose Weight and Feel Great

I Quaderni di Bia

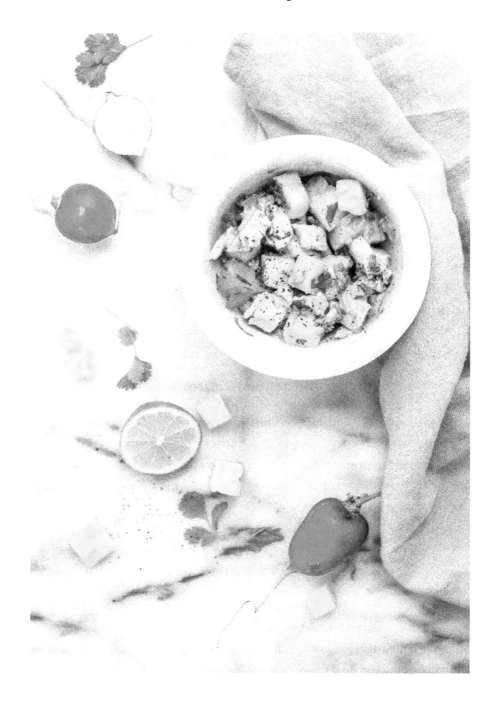

Table of contents

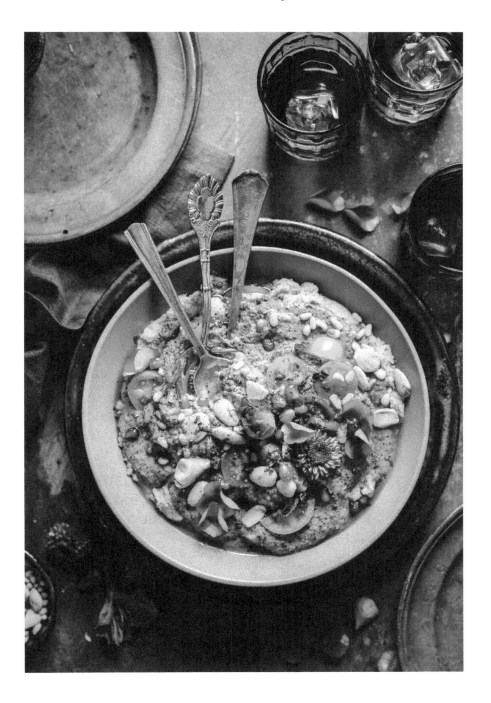

WHAT IS A KETO DiET?

A keto diet is well known for being a low carb diet, where the body produces ketones in the liver to be used as energy. It's referred to as many different names – ketogenic diet, low carb diet, low carb high fat (LCHF), etc.

When you eat something high in carbs, your body will produce glucose and insulin.

Glucose is the easiest molecule for your body to convert and use as energy so that it will be chosen over any other energy source.

Insulin is produced to process the glucose in your bloodstream by taking it around the body.

Since the glucose is being used as a primary energy, your fats are not needed and are therefore stored. Typically on a normal, higher carbohydrate diet, the body will use glucose as the main form of energy. By lowering the intake of carbs, the body is induced into a state known as ketosis.

Ketosis is a natural process the body initiates to help us survive when food intake is low. During this state, we produce ketones, which are produced from the breakdown of fats in the liver.

The end goal of a properly maintained keto diet is to force your body into this metabolic state. We don't do this through starvation of calories but starvation of carbohydrates.

Our bodies are incredibly adaptive to what you put into it – when you overload it with fats and take away carbohydrates, it will begin to burn ketones as the primary energy source. Optimal ketone levels offer many health, weight loss, physical and mental performance benefits.

Benefits of a Ketogenic Diet

There are numerous benefits that come with being on keto: from weight loss and increased energy levels to therapeutic medical applications. Most anyone can safely benefit from eating a low-carb, high-fat diet.

Weight Loss

The ketogenic diet essentially uses your body fat as an energy source – so there are obvious weight loss benefits. On keto, your insulin (the fat storing hormone) levels drop greatly which turns your body into a fat burning machine.

Scientifically, the ketogenic diet has shown better results compared to low-fat and high- carb diets; even in the long term.

Many people incorporate MCT Oil into their diet (it increases ketone production and fat loss) by drinking bulletproof coffee in the morning.

Control Blood Sugar

Keto naturally lowers blood sugar levels due to the type of foods you eat. Studies even show that the ketogenic diet is a more effective way to manage and prevent diabetes compared to low-calorie diets

If you're pre-diabetic or have Type II diabetes, you should seriously consider a ketogenic diet. We have many readers that have had success with their blood sugar control on keto.

Mental Focus

Many people use the ketogenic diet specifically for the increased mental performance.

Ketones are a great source of fuel for the brain. When you lower carb intake, you avoid big spikes in blood sugar. Together, this can result in improved focus and concentration.

Studies show that an increased intake of fatty acids can have impacting benefits to our brain's function.

Increased Energy & Normalized Hunger

By giving your body a better and more reliable energy source, you will feel more energized during the day. Fats are shown to be the most effective molecule to burn as fuel.

On top of that, fat is naturally more satisfying and ends up leaving us in a satiated ("full") state for longer.

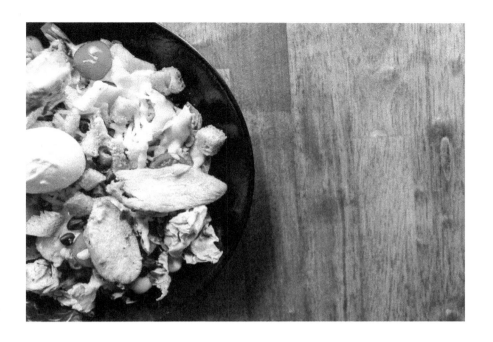

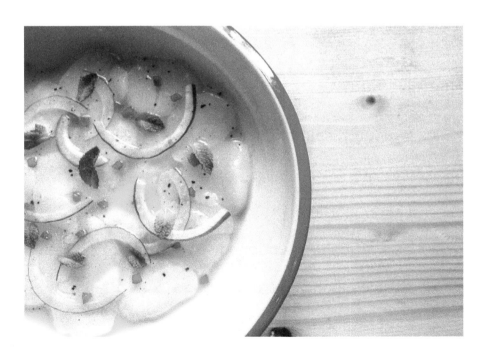

KETOGENIC RECIPES FOR

BREAKFAST

1.Salmon Cakes

This is a Ketogenic breakfast ideayoushouldtrysoon!

Preparation time: 5 minutes

Cooking time: 10 minutes

Servings: 4

Ingredients:

- 1 pound salmonfillets, boneless, skinless and minced
- 1 egg, whisked
- 2 springonions, chopped
- 1 tablespooncilantro, chopped
- 2 tablespoonsalmondflour

- A pinch of salt and black pepper

- 2 tablespoons olive oil

Directions:

1. In a bowl, mix the salmonwith the egg and the otheringredientsexcept the oil, stirwell and shape medium cakes out of this mix.

2. Heat up a pan with the oil over medium heat, add the salmon cakes, cookthemfor 5 minutes on eachside, dividebetween plates and serve for breakfast.

Nutrition:

- Calories 249

- Fat 16.8

- Fiber 0.6

- Carbs 1.4

- Protein 24.3

2.Kale Frittata

Thesewillreallymakeyourdaymucheasier!

Preparation time: 10 minutes

Cooking time: 30 minutes

Servings: 4

Ingredients:

- 8 eggs, whisked 2 shallots, chopped
- 1 tablespoonavocadooil
- 1 cup kale, torn
- Salt and black pepper to the taste
- ¼ cup mozzarella, shredded
- 2 tablespoonschives, chopped

Directions:

1. Heat up a pan with the oil over medium heat, add the shallots, stir and cook for 5minutes.

2. Add the kale, stir and cook for 4 minutes more.

3. Add the eggs mixed with the mozzarella, spread into the pan, sprinkle the chiveson top and bake at 390 degrees F for 20 minutes.

4. Divide the frittatabetween plates and serve.

Nutrition:

- Calories 140

- Fat 6.7

- Fiber 1

- Carbs 4.3

- Protein 10

3.Spinach and Cauliflower Pan

It's a Ketogenic breakfast full of nutrients!

Preparation time: 10 minutes

Cooking time: 18 minutes

Servings: 4

Ingredients:

- 1 pound cauliflowerflorets
- 1 cup baby spinach
- 2 shallots, chopped
- 1 tablespoon olive oil
- 1 tablespoonbalsamicvinegar
- 1 tablespoonparsley, chopped
- ½ cup walnuts, roughlychopped
- Salt and black pepper to the taste

Directions:

1. Heat up a pan with the oil over medium heat, add the shallots, stir and cook for 3minutes.

2. Add the cauliflower and the rest of the ingredients, toss, cook over medium heatfor 15 minutes more, divideinto bowls and serve for breakfast.

Nutrition:

- Calories 140
- Fat 9.3
- Fiber 3
- Carbs 4
- Protein 8

4. Cauliflower Omelet

It's a tastyKetogenicomelet!

Preparation time: 10 minutes

Cooking time: 15 minutes

Servings: 4

Ingredients:

- 4 eggs, whisked 1 cup cauliflowerflorets, chopped 2 springonions, chopped
- 1 tablespoon olive oil
- ½ cup heavycream
- ½ teaspoonsweet paprika
- Salt and black pepper to the taste
- 1 tablespoonchives, chopped

Directions:

1. Heat up a pan with the oil over medium heat, add

the onion and the cauliflower,stir and sauté for 5 minutes.

2. Add the eggs mixed with the cream, paprika, salt and pepper, toss, spread intothe pan, cook over medium heat for 10 minutes, dividebetween plates, sprinklethechives on top and serve.

Nutrition:

- Calories 200
- Fat 4
- Fiber 6
- Carbs 5
- Protein 10

5. Chicken Casserole

It's a savoryKetogenic breakfast you can trytoday!

Preparation time: 10 minutes

Cooking time: 45 minutes

Servings: 4

Ingredients:

- 1 pound chickenbreast, boneless, skinless and ground
- 2 shallots, chopped
- 1 tablespooncoconutoil, melted
- 1 cup baby spinach
- 4 eggs, whisked
- ½ cup parmesan, grated
- Salt and black pepper to the taste
- ½ teaspoongarlicpowder

Directions:

1. Heat up a pan with the oil over medium heat, add the shallots, stir and cook for 5minutes.

2. Add the meat and brown for 5 minutes more.

3. Add the eggs mixed with the garlic and toss.

4. Sprinkle the parmesan on top, introduce in the oven and bake at 390 degreesFfor 35 minutes.

5. Divide the mix between plates and serve.

Nutrition:

- Calories 273
- Fat 13.7
- Fiber 0.2
- Carbs 2.2
- Protein 34.5

6.Spiced Eggs

Try thishealthyketo breakfast reallysoon!

Preparation time: 10 minutes

Cooking time: 15 minutes

Servings: 4

Ingredients:

- 1 tablespoonavocadooil
- 2 springonions, chopped
- 1 tablespooncilantro, chopped
- 4 eggs, whisked
- 1 teaspoon cumin, ground
- 1 teaspoonallspice, ground
- 1 teaspoonnutmeg, ground
- Salt and black pepper to the taste
- 1 tablespoonsparsley, chopped

Directions:

1. Heat up a pan with the oil over medium heat, add the springonions, stirandcook for 2 minutes.

2. Add the eggs and the otheringredients, stir, spread into the pan and cookovermediumheat for 13 minutes.

3. Divide the eggsbetween plates and serve for breakfast.

Nutrition:

- Calories 140
- Fat 6
- Fiber 2
- Carbs 10
- Protein 12

KETOGENIC RECIPES FOR

LUNCH

7.Beef and Radish Stew

It'sdelicious and youwill adore it once youtryit!

Preparation time: 10 minutes

Cooking time: 32 minutes

Servings: 4

Ingredients:

- 1 pound beefstewmeat, cubed
- 2 shallots, chopped
- 2 tablespoons olive oil
- 2 garliccloves, minced
- 1 cup radishes, cubed
- 1 cup black olives, pitted and halved

- 1 cup tomatopassata 1 cup beef stock

- ½ teaspoonrosemary, dried

- ½ teaspoonoregano, dried

- 1 tablespoonparsley, chopped

- A pinch of salt and black pepper

Directions:

1. Heat up a pot with the oil over medium heat, add the shallot and the garlicandsauté for 2 minutes.

2. Add the meat and brown for 5 minutes more.

3. Add the radishes, olives and the otheringredients, bring to a simmer and cookover medium heat for 25 minutes more, stirringoften.

4. Divide the stewinto bowls and serve.

Nutrition:

calories 456 fat 32 fiber 2 carbs 6 protein 30

8. Salmon Bowls

You won't regret tryingthis!

Preparation time: 10 minutes

Cooking time: 15 minutes

Servings: 4

Ingredients:

- 1 pound salmonfillets, boneless, skinless and roughlycubed
- 1 cup chicken stock
- 2 springonions, chopped
- 1 tablespoon olive oil
- 1 cup kalamata olives, pitted and halved
- 1 avocado, pitted, peeled and roughlycubed
- 1 cup baby spinach
- A pinch of salt and black pepper
- ¼ cup cilantro, chopped

- 1 tablespoonbasil, chopped

- 1 teaspoon lime juice

Directions:

1. Heat up a pan with the oil over medium heat, add the springonions and thesalmon, tossgently and cook for 5 minutes.

2. Add the olives and the otheringredients, and cook over medium heat for 10minutes more.

3. Divide the mix into bowls and serve for lunch.

Nutrition:

- Calories 254

- Fat 17

- Fiber 1.9

- Carbs 6.1

- Protein 20

9. Beef and Kale pan

This willreallyget to your soul!

Preparation time: 10 minutes

Cooking time: 20 minutes

Servings: 4

Ingredients:

- 1 pound beefstewmeat, cubed
- 1 redonion, chopped
- 1 tablespoon olive oil
- 2 garliccloves, minced
- 1 cup kale, torn
- 1 cup beef stock
- 1 teaspoon chili powder
- ½ teaspoonsweet paprika
- 1 teaspoonrosemary, dried
- 1 tablespooncilantro, chopped

- A pinch of salt and black pepper

Directions:

1. Heat up a pan with the oil over medium heat, add the onion and the garlic, stirand sauté for 2 minutes.
2. Add the meat and brownit for 5 minutes.
3. Add the rest of the ingredients, bring to a simmer and cook over medium heat for13 minutes more.
4. Divide the mix between plates and serve for lunch.

Nutrition:

- Calories 160
- Fat 10
- Fiber 3
- Carbs 1
- Protein 12

10. Cheesy Pork Casserole

This issomethingyou've been craving for a very long time

Preparation time: 10 minutes

Cooking time: 40 minutes

Servings: 4

Ingredients:

- 1 cup cheddar cheese, grated
- 2 eggs, whisked
- 1 pound pork loin, cubed
- 2 tablespoonsavocadooil
- 2 shallots, chopped
- A pinch of salt and black pepper
- 3 garliccloves, minced
- 1 cup redbellpeppers, cutintostrips

- ¼ cup heavycream

- 1 tablespoonchives, chopped

- ½ teaspoon cumin, ground

Directions:

1. Heat up a pan with the oil over medium heat, add the shallots and the garlicandsauté for 2 minutes.

2. Add the bellpeppers and the meat, toss and cook for 5 minutes more.

3. Add the cumin, salt, pepper, toss and take off the heat.

4. In a bowl, mix the eggswith the cream and the cheese, whisk and pour over thepork mix.

5. Sprinkle the chives on top, introduce the pan in the oven and cook at 380 degreesF for 30 minutes.

6. Divide the mix between plates and serve for lunch.

Nutrition:

- calories 455
- fat 34
- fiber 3
- carbs 3
- protein 33

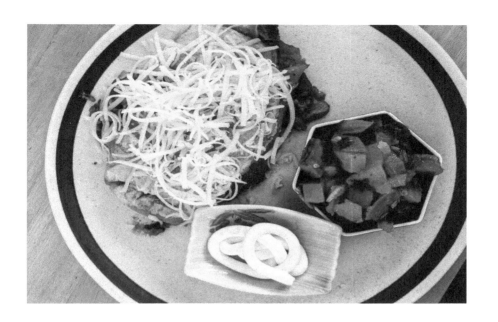

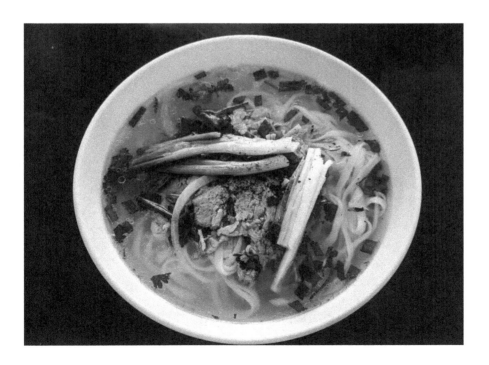

KETOGENIC SIDE DISH

RECIPES

11. Cheesy Tomatoes and Zucchinis

This isrich and flavored!

Preparation time: 10 minutes

Cooking time: 20 minutes

Servings: 4

Ingredients:

- 1 pound cherry tomatoes, halved

- 3 zucchinis, sliced

- 2 tablespoons olive oil

- 1 tablespoonbalsamicvinegar

- 2 garliccloves, minced

- 1 tablespoonoregano, chopped

- A pinch of salt and black pepper

- ½ cup mozzarella, shredded

Directions:

1. In a roasting pan, combine the cherry tomatoeswith the zucchinis and the otheringredientsexcept the mozzarella and toss.

2. Sprinkle the cheese on top, bakeeverything at 400 degrees F for 20 minutes, dividebetween plates and serve as a sidedish.

Nutrition:

- Calories 100

- Fat 2

- Fiber 2

- Carbs 1

- Protein 9

12. Fennel Salad

Preparation time: 10 Servings: 4

Ingredients:

- 2 fennel bulbs, sliced 1 tablespoon lime juice

- 1 tablespoon olive oil ¼ cup walnuts, chopped

- 2 tablespoonschives, chopped

- A pinch of salt and black pepper

Directions:

1. In a bowl, combine the fennelwith the lime juice and the otheringredients, tossandserve as a sidesalad.

Nutrition:

- Calories 80 Fat 0.2 Fiber 1

- Carbs 0.4 Protein 5

13. Spinach and Olives Salad

It's a good idea for a light ketosidedish!

Preparation time: 10 minutes

Cooking time: 12 minutes

Servings: 4

Ingredients:

- ½ pound baby spinach
- 1 cup kalamata olives, pitted and halved
- 1 tablespoon olive oil
- 2 shallots, chopped
- 2 garliccloves, minced
- ½ cup tomatopassata
- 1 tablespooncilantro, chopped
- A pinch of salt and black pepper

Directions:

1. Heat up a pan with the oil over medium heat, add the shallots and garlic, stir and sautéfor 2 minutes.

2. Add the spinach and the otheringredients, toss, cook over medium heat for 10 minutesmore, dividebetween plates and serve.

Nutrition:

- Calories 120
- Fat 3
- Fiber 2
- Carbs 1
- Protein 8

14. Herbed Tomatoes Mix

Wereally like thisketosidedish!

Preparation time: 10 minutes

Cooking time: 30 minutes

Servings: 4

Ingredients:

- 1 pound mixed tomatoes, cutinto wedges

- 2 tablespoons olive oil

- 1 tablespoonoregano, chopped

- 1 tablespoonbasil, chopped

- 1 tablespoonchives, chopped

- 1 tablespoonrosemary, chopped

- 1 tablespoonbalsamicvinegar

- A pinch of salt and black pepper

Directions:

1. In a roasting pan, combine tomatoeswith the oil and the otheringredients, toss and bakeat 380 degrees F for 30 minutes.

2. Divide the tomatoes mix between plates and serve as a sidedish.

Nutrition:

- Calories 150
- Fat 1
- Fiber 2
- Carbs 1
- Protein 8

15. Special Endives And Watercress Side Salad

It'ssuch a freshsidedishthatgoeswith a ketogrilled steak!

Preparation time: 10 minutes Cooking time: 5 minutes Servings: 4

Ingredients:

- 4 medium endives, roots and ends cut and thinlyslicedcrosswise 1 tablespoonlemonjuice
- 1 shallotfinely, chopped 1 tablespoonbalsamicvinegar 2 tablespoons extra virgin olive oil 6 tablespoonsheavycream
- Salt and black pepper to the taste
- 4 ounceswatercress, cut in medium springs
- 1 apple, thinlysliced
- 1 tablespoonchervil, chopped

- 1 tablespoontarragon, chopped

- 1 tablespoonchives, chopped

- 1/3 cup almonds, chopped

- 1 tablespoonparsley, chopped

Directions:

1. In a bowl, mix lemonjuicewithvinegar, salt and shallot, stir and leaveside for 10minutes.

2. Add olive oil, pepper, stir and leaveaside for another 2 minutes.

3. Put endives, apple, watercress, chives, tarragon, parsley and chervil in a salad bowl.

4. Addsalt and pepper to the taste and toss to coat.

5. Addheavycream and vinaigrette, stirgently and serve as a sidedishwithalmondsontop.

Nutrition:

Calories 200 Fat 3 Fiber 5 Carbs 2 Protein 10

16.   Indian Side Salad

It'sveryhealthy and rich!

Preparation time: 15 minutes

Cooking time: 0 minutes

Servings: 6

Ingredients:

- 3 carrots, finelygrated
- 2 courgettes, finelysliced
- A bunch of radishes, finelysliced
- ½ redonion, chopped
- 6 mintleaves, roughlychopped
- For the salad dressing:
- 1 teaspoonmustard
- 1 tablespoonshomemade mayo
- 1 tablespoonsbalsamicvinegar
- 2 tablespoons extra virgin olive oil

- Salt and black pepper to the taste

Directions:

1. In a bowl, mix mustardwith mayo, vinegar, salt and pepper to the taste and stirwell.
2. Addoilgradually and whisk everything.
3. In a salad bowl, mix carrotswithradishes, courgettes and mintleaves.
4. Addsalad dressing, toss to coat and keep in the fridgeuntilyou serve it.

Nutrition:

- Calories 140
- Fat 1
- Fiber 2
- Carbs 1
- Protein 7

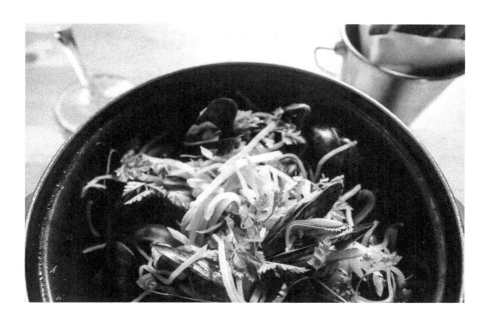

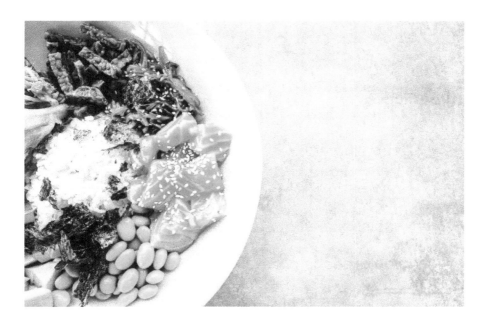

KETOGENIC SNACKS AND

APPETIZERS RECIPES

17.   Nuts and Seed Bowls

This is a greatketo snack for a casual day!

Preparation time: 5 minutes

Cooking time: 20 minutes

Servings: 6

Ingredients:

- 1 cup walnuts

- 1 cup almonds

- 1 tablespoonsunflowerseeds

- 2 tablespoons olive oil

- A pinch of salt and black pepper

- ½ teaspoonsweet paprika

Directions:

1. In a bowl, mix the walnutswith the almonds, seeds and the otheringredients,toss and spread on a bakingsheetlinedwithparchmentpaper.

2. Bake at 400 degrees F for 20 minutes, divideinto bowls and serve as a snack.

Nutrition:

- Calories 140
- Fat 2
- Fiber 1
- Carbs 5
- Protein 1

18. TomatoDip

Try thistoday!

Preparation time: 10 minutes

Cooking time: 15 minutes

Servings: 4

Ingredients:

- 1 cup creamcheese, soft
- ¼ cup tomatopassata
- 1 tablespoonbasil, chopped
- ½ teaspoonsweet paprika
- Salt and black pepper to the taste

Directions:

1. In a bowl, combine the creamcheesewith the passata and the otheringredients,whisk well,

divideinto 4 ramekins, introduce in the oven at 370 degrees F andbake for 15 minutes.

2. Serve cold.

Nutrition:

- Calories 140

- Fat 4

- Fiber 2

- Carbs 6

- Protein 4

19.   **Zucchini Salsa**

Enjoy a greatappetizer right away!

Preparation time: 10 minutes Cooking time: 12 minutes Servings: 6

Ingredients:

- 3 zucchinis, roughlycubed
- 3 springonions, chopped
- 1 cup black olives, pitted and halved
- 1 cup cherry tomatoes, halved
- Salt and black pepper to the taste
- 2 tablespoons olive oil
- 2 tablespoonsbalsamicvinegar

Directions:

1. Heat up a pan with the oil over medium heat, add the springonions and thezucchinis, stir and sauté

for 2 minutes.

2. Add the rest of the ingredients, toss, cook for 10 minutes more, divideintobowlsand serve cold.

Nutrition:

- Calories 40
- Fat 3
- Fiber 7
- Carbs 3
- Protein 7

20.   Leeks Hummus

Everyone loves a good hummus! Try this one!

Preparation time: 5 minutes

Cooking time: 0 minutes

Servings: 4

Ingredients:

- 4 leeks, chopped

- ¼ cup avocadooil

- Salt and black pepper to the taste

- 4 garliccloves, minced

- 1 cup sesameseeds paste

- 2 tablespoons lime juice

- 1 tablespoonchives, chopped

Directions:

1. In your blender, mix the leekswith the oil, salt,

pepper and the otheringredients,pulse well, divideinto bowls and serve cold.

Nutrition:

- Calories 80
- Fat 5
- Fiber 3
- Carbs 6
- Protein 7

21. Chicken Dip

Preparation time: 6 minutes

Cooking time: 0 minutes

Servings: 8

Ingredients:

- 2 cups rotisseriechicken, skinless, bonelessshredded
- 2 redchilies, minced
- 2 springonions, chopped
- ¼ cup creamcheese, soft
- Salt and black pepper to the taste
- ½ teaspoonsmoked paprika

Directions:

1. In a bowl, combine the chickenwith the chilies and the otheringredients, stirwell,

divideintosmall bowls and serve as a party dip.

Nutrition:

- Calories 100

- Fat 2

- Fiber 3

- Carbs 1

- Protein 6

KETOGENIC FISH AND

SEAFOOD RECIPES

22.   Shrimp and Fennel

You should consider making this for dinner tonight!

Preparation time: 5 minutes

Cooking time: 10 minutes

Servings: 4

Ingredients:

- 1 pound big shrimp, peeled and deveined

- 1 fennel bulb, sliced

- ¼ cup chicken stock

- 2 tablespoons olive oil

- Juice of 1 lime

- A pinch of salt and black pepper

- 1 teaspoon sweet paprika

- 1 teaspoon allspice

- 1 tablespoon cilantro, chopped

Directions:

1. Heat up a pan with the oil over medium heat, add the fennel and cook it for 3minutes.

2. Add the shrimp and the other ingredients, cook over medium heat for 7 minutesmore, divide into bowls and serve.

Nutrition:

- Calories 120

- Fat 3

- Fiber 1

- Carbs 2

- Protein 6

23. Shrimp and Salmon Pan

Have you ever tried something like this?

Preparation time: 10 minutes

Cooking time: 15 minutes

Servings: 4

Ingredients:

- 2 tablespoons avocado oil

- 3 shallots, minced

- 1 garlic clove, minced

- 1 pound shrimp, peeled and deveined

- ½ pound salmon fillets, boneless, skinless and cubed

- ½ cup tomato passata

- ¼ cup cilantro, chopped

- A pinch of salt and black pepper

Directions:

1. Heat up a pan with the oil over medium heat, add the shallots and the garlic andsauté for 2 minutes.
2. Add the salmon and cook for 3 minutes more.
3. Add the shrimp and the other ingredients, cook over medium heat for 10 minutesmore, divide into bowls and serve.

Nutrition:

- Calories 250
- Fat 12
- Fiber 3
- Carbs 5
- Protein 20

24. Shrimp and Mushroom Mix

Preparation time: 10 minutes

Cooking time: 15 minutes

Servings: 4

Ingredients:

- ½ pound baby bell mushrooms, sliced
- 1 pound shrimp, peeled and deveined
- 2 tablespoons olive oil
- A pinch of salt and black pepper
- 1 teaspoon red pepper flakes, crushed
- 2 garlic cloves, minced
- 1 cup heavy cream

Directions:

1. Heat up a pan with the oil over medium heat, add

the garlic and the pepper flakesand cook for 2 minutes

2. Add the mushrooms, toss and cook for 5 minutes more.

3. Add the shrimp and the other ingredients, toss, cook over medium heat for 8minutes more, divide into bowls and serve.

Nutrition:

- Calories 455

- Fat 6

- Fiber 5

- Carbs 4

- Protein 13

25. Shrimp and Ginger Mix

It's one of the best ways to enjoy some shrimp!

Preparation time: 10 minutes

Cooking time: 10 minutes Servings: 4

Ingredients:

- 2 spring onions, chopped
- 2 tablespoons coconut oil, melted
- 1 tablespoon ginger, grated
- 2 tablespoons coconut aminos
- 1 pound shrimp, peeled and deveined
- A pinch of salt and black pepper
- ½ tablespoon chives, chopped

Directions:

1. Heat up a pot with the oil over medium heat, add

the spring onions and theginger and cook for 2 minutes.

2. Add the shrimp and the other ingredients, toss, cook for 8 minutes more, divideinto bowls and serve.

Nutrition:

- Calories 200

- Fat 3

- Fiber 2

- Carbs 4

- Protein 14

26. Calamari and Ghee Mix

You only need some simple ingredients to make this!

Preparation time: 5 minutes

Cooking time: 20 minutes Servings: 4

Ingredients:

- 1 pound calamari rings
- ½ cup chicken stock
- 2 garlic cloves, minced
- 2 tablespoons ghee, melted
- 2 tablespoons lime juice
- 1 tablespoon parsley, chopped

Directions:

1. Heat up a pan with the ghee over medium heat, add the garlic and cook for 1minute.

2. Add the calamari and the other ingredients, toss, cook over medium heat for 18minutes more, divide into bowls and serve.

Nutrition:

- Calories 50
- Fat 1
- Fiber 0
- Carbs 0.5
- Protein 2

27.   **Basil Tuna**

This is one of our favorite keto dishes!

Preparation time: 10 minutes

Cooking time: 14 minutes Servings: 4

Ingredients:

- 4 tuna fillets, boneless

- 2 tablespoons olive oil

- 1 tablespoon basil, chopped

- 2 spring onions, chopped

- A pinch of salt and black pepper

- A pinch of cayenne pepper

- 1 tablespoons garlic, minced

Directions:

1. Heat up a pan with the oil medium heat, add the spring onions and the garlic andcook for 2

minutes more.

2. Add the tuna and the other ingredients, cook the fish for 5 minutes on each side,divide between plates and serve.

Nutrition:

- Calories 345

- Fat 32

- Fiber 3

- Carbs 3

- Protein 13

KETOGENIC POULTRY

RECIPES

28. Chicken and Zucchini Casserole

This could be your lunch today!

Preparation time: 10 minutes

Cooking time: 40 minutes

Servings: 4

Ingredients:

- 2 pounds chicken breast, skinless and boneless and sliced

- 2 tablespoons olive oil

- 2 spring onions, chopped

- 2 zucchinis, roughly cubed

- A pinch of salt and black pepper

- 1 teaspoon oregano, dried

- 1 teaspoon basil, dried

- 1 cup tomato passata

- 1 cup parmesan, grated

- 1 tablespoon parsley, chopped

Directions:

1. Heat up a pan with the oil over medium high heat, add the spring onions andsauté for 2 minutes.

2. Add the chicken and cook for 2 minutes on each side.

3. Transfer this to a baking dish, add the zucchinis and the other ingredients exceptthe cheese and the parsley.

4. Sprinkle the cheese and the parsley on top, introduce the oven and bake at 375degrees F for 35 minutes.

5. Divide the mix between plates and serve.

Nutrition:

- Calories 300
- Fat 6
- Fiber 3
- Carbs 5
- Protein 28

29. Chicken and Cauliflower

These will really impress your guests!

Preparation time: 10 minutes

Cooking time: 30 minutes

Servings: 4

Ingredients:

- 2 cups cauliflower florets
- 1 pound chicken breast, skinless, boneless and cubed
- 2 tablespoons olive oil
- 2 shallots, chopped
- A pinch of salt and black pepper
- 1 cup chicken stock
- 1 teaspoon sweet paprika
- 1 cup mozzarella, shredded

Directions:

1. Heat up a pan with the oil over medium heat, add the shallots and sauté for 5minutes.
2. Add the chicken and brown for 5 minutes more.
3. Add the rest of the ingredients except the cheese and toss gently.
4. Sprinkle the cheese on top, introduce in the oven at 350 degrees F and bake for20 minutes.
5. Divide everything between plates and serve.

Nutrition:

- Calories 200
- Fat 6
- Fiber 3
- Carbs 6
- Protein 14

30. Chicken and Garlic Green Beans

This is a really delicious keto chicken dish!

Preparation time: 10 minutes

Cooking time: 30 minutes

Servings: 4

Ingredients:

- 1 pound chicken breast, skinless and boneless and roughly cubed
- 2 tablespoons avocado oil
- 2 shallots, chopped
- ½ pound green beans, trimmed and halved
- 4 garlic cloves, mined
- 1 cup chicken stock
- ½ cup tomato passata
- 1 tablespoon cilantro, chopped

- A pinch of salt and black pepper

Directions:

1. Heat up a pan with the oil over medium heat, add the shallots and the meat andbrown for 5 minutes.

2. Add the garlic and the green beans, and cook for 5 minutes more.

3. Add the rest of the ingredients, toss gently, bring to a simmer and cook overmedium heat for 20 minutes more.

4. Divide between plates and serve.

Nutrition:

- Calories 240 Fat 4
- Fiber 3
- Carbs 6
- Protein 20

31.   Chicken and Broccoli Casserole

You must really make this tonight!

Preparation time: 10 minutes

Cooking time: 35 minutes

Servings: 4

Ingredients:

- 1 pound chicken breasts, skinless, boneless, cubed
- 2 tablespoons olive oil
- 2 cups broccoli florets
- 1 teaspoon smoked paprika
- 1 teaspoon rosemary, dried
- 1 teaspoon oregano, dried
- 1 cup chicken stock
- 1 cup parmesan, grated

- A pinch of salt and black pepper

Directions:

1. Heat up a pan with the oil over medium heat, add the chicken and brown it for 5minutes.

2. Transfer this to a baking dish, add the broccoli and the other ingredients exceptthe cheese and toss.

3. Sprinkle the cheese on top, introduce the pan in the oven and bake at 370 degreesF for 30 minutes

4. Divide between plates and serve.

Nutrition:

- Calories 250 Fat 5

- Fiber 4

- Carbs 6

- Protein 25

32. Chicken, Tomatoes and Green Beans

The taste is so amazing!

Preparation time: 10 minutes

Cooking time: 35 minutes

Servings: 4

Ingredients:

- 2 tablespoons olive oil

- 1 pound chicken breast, skinless, boneless and cubed

- 1 cup cherry tomatoes, halved

- 1 celery stalks, chopped

- ½ pound green beans, trimmed and halved

- 1 cup tomato passata

- 1 cup mozzarella, shredded

- A pinch of salt and black pepper

- 1 tablespoon cilantro, chopped

Directions:

1. Heat up a pan with the oil over medium heat, add the chicken and the celery andcook for 5 minutes.
2. Add the green beans and the other ingredients except the cheese, toss and cookfor 5 minutes more.
3. Sprinkle the cheese on top, introduce in the oven and bake at 380 degrees F for25 minutes.
4. Divide the mix between plates and serve.

Nutrition:

- Calories 400 Fat 23
- Fiber 5
- Carbs 5
- Protein 30

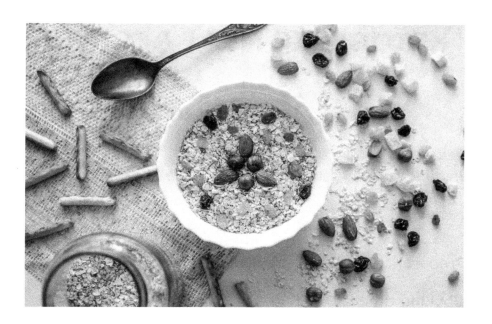

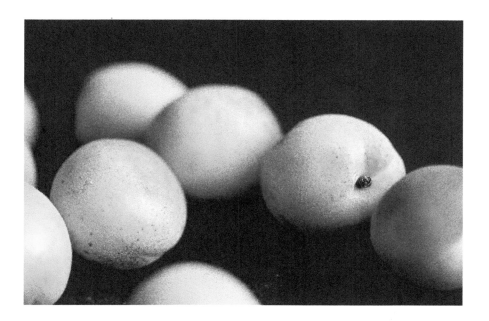

KETOGENIC MEAT RECIPES

33.   Marjoram Beef

It only takes a few minutes to make this special keto recipe!

Preparation time: 10 minutes

Cooking time: 30 minutes

Servings: 4

Ingredients:

- 1 pound beef stew meat, cubed
- 2 tablespoons ghee, melted
- 1 red onion, chopped
- 2 garlic cloves, minced
- 1 cup beef stock
- 2 teaspoons sweet paprika
- 1 tablespoon marjoram, chopped

- A pinch of salt and black pepper

Directions:

1. Heat up a pan with the ghee over medium heat, add the onion and the garlic and sauté for 5minutes.
2. Add the meat and brown for 5 minutes more.
3. Add the rest of the ingredients, bring to a simmer and cook over medium heat for 20 minutesmore.
4. Divide everything into bowls and serve.

Nutrition:

- Calories 320
- Fat 13
- Fiber 4
- Carbs 12
- Protein 40

34.   Spiced Beef

This is really tasty! You must make it for your family tonight!

Preparation time: 10 minutes

Cooking time: 35 minutes

Servings: 4

Ingredients:

- 3 garlic cloves, minced
- 2 pounds beef stew meat, cubed
- ½ cup beef stock
- 2 tablespoons avocado oil
- 2 chilii peppers, chopped
- 1 teaspoon thyme, dried
- ½ teaspoon coriander, ground
- ½ teaspoon allspice, ground
- 2 teaspoons cumin, ground

- ½ teaspoon turmeric powder

- ¼ teaspoon nutmeg, ground

- A pinch of salt and black pepper

- 1 teaspoon garlic powder

Directions:

1. Heat up a pan with the oil over medium heat, add the garlic and the meat and brown for 5minutes.

2. Add the thyme, coriander and the rest of the ingredients, toss, bring to a simmer and cook overmedium heat for 30 minutes more.

3. Divide everything between plates and serve.

Nutrition:

- Calories 267 Fat 23

- Fiber 1

- Carbs 3

- Protein 12

KETOGENIC VEGETABLE

RECIPES

35. Asparagus and Tomatoes

It'sreally, reallytasty!

Preparation time: 10 minutes

Cooking time: 20 minutes

Servings: 4

Ingredients:

- ¼ cup shallots, chopped

- 2 tablespoons olive oil

- 4 asparagus spears, trimmed and halved

- 1 pound cherry tomatoes, halved

- A pinch of salt and black pepper

- 1 cup cheddar cheese, grated

Directions:

1. In a roasting pan, combine the asparagus with the shallots and the otheringredients, tossandbake at 400 degrees F for 20 minutes.
2. Divide the mix between plates and serve.

Nutrition:

- Calories 200
- Fat 12
- Fiber 2
- Carbs 5
- Protein 14

36. Endives and Mustard Sauce

It's a verycreamyketodishyou can trytonight!

Preparation time: 10 minutes

Cooking time: 20 minutes

Servings: 4

Ingredients:

- 2 endives, trimmed and halvedlengthwise
- 2 tablespoons olive oil 2 shallots, chopped
- A pinch of salt and black pepper
- 2 tablespoons parmesan, grated
- 2 tablespoonsmustard
- ¼ cup heavycream

Directions:

1. Heat up a pan with the oil over medium heat, add

the shallots and sauté for 2 minutes.

2. Add the endives and the otheringredientsexcept the parmesan, toss, and cook over medium heatfor 15 minutes more.

3. Add the parmesan, toss, cookeverything for 3 minutes more, dividebetween plates and serve.

Nutrition:

- Calories 256

- Fat 23

- Fiber 2

- Carbs 5

- Protein 13

37. Baked Brussels Sprouts

This issofresh and full of vitamins! It'swonderful!

Preparation time: 10 minutes

Cooking time: 20 minutes

Servings: 4

Ingredients:

- 1 pound Brussels sprouts, trimmed and halved
- 1 tablespoonavocadooil 2 garliccloves, minced
- A pinch of salt and black pepper
- ¼ cup cilantro, chopped

Directions:

1. In a roasting pan, combine the sproutswith the oil and the otheringredients, toss and bake at 400degrees F for 20 minutes.

2. Divideeverythingbetween plates and serve.

Nutrition:

- Calories 100

- Fat 3

- Fiber 1

- Carbs 2

- Protein 6

38.   Roasted Tomatoes

If youdon't have time to cook a complexdinnertonight,

thentrythis!

Preparation time: 10 minutes

Cooking time: 25 minutes

Servings: 4

Ingredients:

- 1 pound tomatoes, halved

- A pinch of salt and black pepper

- 2 tablespoons olive oil 1 teaspoonrosemary, dried 1 teaspoonbasil, dried

- 1 tablespoonchives, chopped

Directions:

1. In a roasting pan combine the tomatoeswith the oil and the otheringredients, tossgentlyandbake

at 390 degrees F for 25 minutes.

2. Divide the mix between plates and serve.

Nutrirtion:

- Calories 122

- Fat 12

- Fiber 1

- Carbs 3

- Protein 14

39.   Brussels Sprouts and

Green Beans

Do youwant to learn how to makethistastyketodish?.

Preparation time: 10 minutes

Cooking time: 20 minutes Servings: 4

Ingredients:

- 1 tablespoonavocadooil

- 1 pound Brussels sprouts, trimmed and halved

- ½ pound green beans, trimmed and halved

- ½ teaspoongarlicpowder

- A pinch of salt and black pepper

- 1 tablespoon lime juice

Directions:

1. In a roasting pan, combine the sproutswith the

   green   beans   and   the   otheringredients,

toss,introduce in the oven at 375 degrees F and bake for 20 minutes.

2. Dividebetween plates and serve.

Nutrition:

- Calories 80
- Fat 5
- Fiber 2
- Carbs 5
- Protein 7

KETOGENIC DESSERT

RECIPES

40.   Cinnamon Cream

You must trythisspecial mix as well!

Preparation time: 2 hours

Cooking time: 10 minutes Servings: 4

Ingredients:

- 2 tablespoonsswerve 1 cup coconutmilk

- 1 cup heavycream

- 1 tablespooncinnamonpowder

- ¼ teaspoonginger, ground

Directions:

1. In a bowl, combine the creamwith the milk and

the otheringredients, whisk well, transfer to apot, heat up over medium heat for 10 minutes and divideinto bowls.

2. Keep in the fridge for 2 hoursbeforeserving.

Nutrition:

- Calories 244

- Fat 25.4

- Fiber 1.3

- Carbs 5.2

- Protein 2